Daniel Fernando Magrini

Nursing, its attitudes and behaviour towards suicide

Daniel Fernando Magrini

Nursing, its attitudes and behaviour towards suicide

Attitudes of nursing professionals working in emergencies towards suicidal behaviour and associated factors

ScienciaScripts

Imprint
Any brand names and product names mentioned in this book are subject to trademark, brand or patent protection and are trademarks or registered trademarks of their respective holders. The use of brand names, product names, common names, trade names, product descriptions etc. even without a particular marking in this work is in no way to be construed to mean that such names may be regarded as unrestricted in respect of trademark and brand protection legislation and could thus be used by anyone.

Cover image: www.ingimage.com

This book is a translation from the original published under ISBN 978-613-9-63832-1.

Publisher:
Sciencia Scripts
is a trademark of
Dodo Books Indian Ocean Ltd. and OmniScriptum S.R.L publishing group

120 High Road, East Finchley, London, N2 9ED, United Kingdom
Str. Armeneasca 28/1, office 1, Chisinau MD-2012, Republic of Moldova, Europe
Printed at: see last page
ISBN: 978-620-7-70305-0

I dedicate this dissertation and everything it represents to my wife Amanda and my son Luigi. In addition to my smile, God will give you back my gratitude in happiness for our family.

Thank you

I would like to thank my supervisor, Prof Dr Kelly Graziani Giacchero Vedana, for her guidance and for being part of this scientific construction. As well as being a teacher, I'm sure she was humane, fair and understanding.

To my family and my parents, who taught me values that have helped me realise today that something material should not take precedence over something spiritual.

To the teachers of all the subjects I took during my master's degree and the teaching improvement programme.

To nurse Miyeko Hayashida for her considerations during the qualifying exam and in setting up the database. To statistician Jonas Bodini Alonso for his guidance and availability and to librarian Mr Robson Araújo for his considerations on technical standards.

To Thatiana Guioto who introduced me to Professor Kelly, to Eliana Arantes who encouraged me to continue studying and to Victor Hugo and Marina Gifali for their contribution to data collection.

To the Ribeirão Preto School of Nursing for welcoming me and to the staff of the postgraduate secretariat who were always on hand.

To the hospital and SAMU services and all the professionals who took part in the research.

To the members of the examining board.

The Centre for Psychosocial Care III (CAPS III), my place of work, because it contributed greatly to my work and study day.

"What is essential is invisible to the eye. You can only truly love with your heart."

Antoine de Saint-Exupéry

SUMMARY

MAGRINI, D. F. M. Attitudes of nursing professionals working in emergencies towards suicidal behaviour and associated factors. 2016. 83 f. Dissertation (Master's) - Ribeirão Preto School of Nursing, University of São Paulo, Ribeirão Preto, 2016.

Suicide is a preventable problem with a significant global impact. Nursing professionals who work in emergency departments play a central role n the initial management of suicide attempts and the quality of care provided by these professionals can be influenced by their attitudes towards suicidal behaviour. Knowledge about attitudes towards suicide and associated factors is scarce and needs to be investigated in different countries, cultures and times. This study investigated attitudes towards suicide and associated factors among nursing professionals working in emergency departments. This is a quantitative cross-sectional study carried out with a population of 146 nursing professionals from two emergency services (pre-hospital and hospital) in the interior of São Paulo, Brazil. Data was collected in 2015 by self-applying a sociodemographic questionnaire and the Questionnaire of Attitudes towards Suicidal Behaviour (QACS). This questionnaire has no cut-off points and can be analysed using the individual items and the factors *"Feelings towards the patient"*, *"Perception of professional capacity" and "Right to suicide"*. The data was analysed using the Statistical Package for the Social Sciences (SPSS) software, version 19.0 and R GUI 3.0.1. The Kolmogorov-Smirnova and Shapiro-Wilk normality tests, the Spearman correlation test and the Mann-Whitney test were applied. The participants had low educational exposure to suicide and the minimum and maximum scores on each of the questionnaire items were obtained. More negative attitudes were associated with having worked in a mental health service (p=0.00). Greater perception of professional ability was associated with specific training in mental health (p=0.00) or suicide (p=0.00) and working in a hospital service (p=0.01). Less moralistic and condemnatory attitudes were associated with experience of working in mental health services (p=0.01) and being a nurse (p=0.00). There was a weak positive correlation between perceived professional ability and less negative attitudes. This study is a pioneer in the investigation of factors associated with attitudes towards suicide among nursing professionals who work in emergencies in the Brazilian hospital and pre-hospital context. It is important to invest in strategies that promote the mental health of professionals, better attitudes and preparation for the qualification of care.

Keywords: Suicide; Suicide attempt; Nursing; Attitude.

SUMMARY

Presentation

During secondary school, I studied building trades to become a master builder, but I didn't want to pursue this career. I decided to take a nursing assistant course in parallel and then a nursing technician course when I was 18. A year after graduating, I passed the public examination in nursing and started working. At the hospital, I learnt about other professions and thought about continuing my studies.

In 2004, I started my Bachelor's Degree in Psychology while working at the hospital. A friend of mine in Neurosurgery was doing "a kind of scientific initiation" and asked if I would like to do an internship there with Professor Dr Sílvio Morato. He welcomed me into the Psychobiology laboratory and, after two years, I completed my research with Wistar rats. I was invited to do a master's degree in that area, but I used emotion more than reason and gave up on that field, as I wanted the opportunity to research human beings. This decision cost me to start from scratch and I ended up focussing on competitions for psychologists. So I gave up the idea of starting a postgraduate course.

When I went to work in the field of mental health, I still felt a void and commented on it to one of Professor Kelly's students who said she would introduce her to me. Maybe there was something I could contribute and get closer to the academic field. Science has always fascinated me because I'm very curious, I like to talk and I like to listen.

Professor Kelly welcomed me with open arms. At the time, I didn't intend to do a master's degree, I just wanted to do research. I helped with data collection, interviews and analyses using the methodology of Grounded Theory.

When the idea of a master's degree became part of our conversations, I thought it would be interesting and important to do some research into suicide. The gap in knowledge led us to research the meanings and attitudes of nursing professionals who work in emergencies. I deal with suicidal patients every day in my workplace and I know what the teams go through, so demonstrating this scientifically is fair and important.

I took part in the selection process to study for a master's degree at the Ribeirão Preto School of Nursing and was approved. I realised that a whole world had opened up before me. There is a reality that few people know about, which is the scientific world. In a scientific initiation we don't have the chance to feel the pulse of the disciplines, the organisation, the demands, to get to know teaching more closely.

I overcame many blockages that a life of difficulties had deeply engraved in me and today I know that I've come very little way in the academic field, but I know that nothing is impossible and that with dedication, opportunities and good guidance (and by good I mean guidance with the soul), we can go to infinity.

Today I'm defending a master's degree, and as I told my supervisor, I wanted it to be the best. I hope it was, at least I tried to make it so. My gratitude won't only be returned through published articles or a good grade in the subjects. I don't know where I'll end up, but I'll always be grateful to everyone who has contributed to this journey.

I am therefore presenting this dissertation entitled "Attitudes of nursing professionals working in emergencies towards suicidal behaviour and associated factors", with the aim of providing academia with relevant information about these attitudes towards suicidal behaviour. The results could therefore contribute to the technical and attitudinal aspects of nursing teams working in urgent and emergency care centres and dealing with suicide.

CHAPTER 1

Introduction

Suicide is an enigmatic, complex phenomenon that is difficult to rationalise, understand or explain. However, it is highly frequent, impactful, underestimated and taboo in today's society.

Suicide can be defined as self-induced death, which has sufficient evidence (explicit or implicit) to allow the deduction that the person's wish was to die (DE LEO et aL, 2006; EMERGENCY NURSES ASSOCIATION - ENA, 2012; NANTON, 2014; SILVERMAN et aL, 2007). It is important to understand definitions related to suicidal behaviour.

Suicide has a broader definition than suicide, as it includes any act in which an individual causes injury to themselves, whatever the degree of lethal intent and knowledge of the real reason for the act. Suicidal behaviour ranges from thoughts of self-destruction, threats, gestures, suicide attempts to completed suicide (WERLANG; BOTEGA, 2004).

Suicidal behaviour can be observed along a *continuum, that* is, with conditions that precede the act of suicide, in which the person initially has thoughts of self-destruction, which can be followed by threats, gestures, which lead to suicide attempts (WORLD HEALTH ORGANIZATION - WHO, 2014).

Such attempts are defined as self-injurious behaviour with non-fatal consequences, accompanied by evidence (explicit or implicit) that the person intended to die.

In addition to the terms mentioned above, there are other definitions related to suicidology (the science that studies suicide), which contribute to understanding the wide variety of suicidal behaviours (CASSORLA, 2004).

- Parasuicide: a suicidal act without a fatal outcome, regardless of how serious the act was medically or psychologically;

- Unconscious suicides: all acts that contribute to an individual's death, even if the intention was not to kill themselves. Examples include traffic accidents, "accidental" poisoning, accidents in the home, at work, unnecessary exposure to dangers such as the use of illicit drugs or the simple act of going without food;

- Anniversary reactions: these are pathological phenomena involving psychological, social, cultural and mental factors, which occur around or on the date of the death of a loved one. It can occur, for example, when the suicidal person reaches the age of the loved one who died. They are considered a form of pathological bereavement;

- Homicide precipitated by the victim: in this case the victim encourages someone to kill them, either gradually or completely, so it is a self-destructive condition that requires the help of a third party;

- Unconscious fantasies: these are those in which the individual apparently does not have the aim of dying, but rather to change their situation, often with the aim of escaping suffering or finding a reward after the act. For example, some unconscious fantasies that could justify suicidal acts are: killing oneself to find another life or a paradise world, revenge, reunion or self-punishment and asking for help;

- Altruistic suicide: occurs in defence of other individuals or some ideal, for example, hunger strikes, protests, blowing up planes at enemies.

There are different perspectives from which suicidal behaviour can be analysed. The sociological perspective considers that society plays an important role in the occurrence of suicide. In this way, it is assumed that each act of suicide should not be observed in isolation, as it has its own eminently social nature (DURKHEIN, 1982).

Among different religious beliefs, there are variations between punishments and rewards for suicidal behaviour. But in general, suicide is considered a wrong and reprehensible act (JUNG; OLSON, 2014). Psychology has different models and hypotheses that seek to understand this behaviour. There are also legal issues related to suicide, which is considered a crime in some countries, unlike Brazil.

Suicide is a multifaceted and particularly challenging problem in clinical practice. It is a multidimensional phenomenon and is associated with biological, genetic, psychological and sociological factors (BERG, 2016; SUN, et aL, 2015; ZADRAVEC; GRAD, 2013).

It is understood that there are protective factors, predisposing factors and more recent precipitating factors, such as unemployment, social crises, the break-up of a romantic relationship (BERG, 2016; BOTEGA, 2016).

Individual risk factors for suicide include physical illness, mental disorders, specific psychiatric symptoms (anxiety, hopelessness, impulsiveness and aggressiveness), previous psychiatric history of physical or sexual abuse in childhood, psychosocial stressors, family history of suicide (QUEVEDO; SCHMITT; KAPCZINSKI, 2008). Lack of social support also seems to be a relevant factor, since suicide is more prevalent among people who are alone or have few friends (GOUDA; RAO, 2008).

Previous suicide attempts are the main risk factor for future suicide (OWENS; HORROCKS;

HOUSE, 2002), and the person's risk of committing the act increases according to the number of attempts and is also linked to the minimum time gap between these attempts (BERTOLOTE et aL, 2010; QUEVEDO; SCHMITT; KAPCZINSKI 2008; VIDAL, GONTIJO, 2013).

It must be taken into account that social situations and issues such as employability, family structure, lack of jobs, socio-economic conditions, the standard of possibilities for consuming inputs, acceptance in the environment, among other factors, also interfere with suicidal behaviour (WORLD HEALTH ORGANISATION - WHO, 2002).

The motives associated with attempted self-harm are diverse and can include the desire to cause one's own death, avoid psychological suffering or an intolerable situation, influence changes in behaviour, test people's feelings about them, provoke feelings of pity and guilt, show despair, seek help, among others (QUEVEDO; SCHMITT; KAPCZINSKI, 2008). Regardless of the real intention of the person aware of the lethality of the method, there is an expression of suffering or dysfunctional behaviour associated with self-injury.

Suicide usually symbolises the search for a solution to a problem, a crisis that generates suffering. It is also linked to unmet needs, feelings of hopelessness, despair and helplessness, conflicts between survival and unbearable stress, narrowing of alternatives and the search for escape, in other words, situations in which the suicidal person shows signs of distress (KAPLAN, SADOCK, GREBB, 2002). Given the complexity of suicidal behaviour, prevention efforts should be based on modifiable risk factors and protective factors (BOTEGA, 2014).

Suicide is the second leading cause of death among people aged 15 to 29 (WHO, 2014). There are also at least five or six people linked to the suicide who are deeply affected emotionally, socially and economically (WHO, 2008; CARMONA-NAVARRO; PICHARDO-MARTÍNEZ, 2012).

It is estimated that in 2012 there were 804,000 deaths by suicide worldwide, representing an annual rate of 11.4 suicides per 100,000 inhabitants, one death every 40 seconds (WHO, 2014), and the projection for 2020 is at least 1.53 million deaths (VOLPE, CORRÊA, BARRERO, 2006). More people commit suicide every year than die in all the world's conflicts combined (WHO, 2006).

Brazil ranks eighth in absolute numbers of suicides. In the municipality of Campinas in 2003, a study found that 17.1 per cent of people had "seriously thought about ending their lives", 4.8 per cent had death plans and 2.8 per cent had attempted suicide (BOTEGA et aL, 2009).

Suicide attempts reach high rates and can be ten or 20 times the number of completed suicides (BERTOLOTE et aL, 2010; WHO, 2014). Lifetime prevalence rates for suicide attempts range from 0.4% to 4.2% (VIDAL, GONTIJO, 2013). Suicide attempts are more common in women, while completed suicide is more common in men (BERTOLOTE et aL, 2010).

Due to the increase in the number of suicides, as well as the associated damage, the World Health Organisation recommends that the problem be prioritised on health and public policy agendas (WHO, 2014).

In Brazil, considering the seriousness and the possibility of prevention, the Ministry of Health launched Ordinance No. 1,876 in 2006, which establishes National Guidelines for Suicide Prevention and emphasises the importance of research on the subject (BRASIL, 2006).

Qualified assessment and intervention regarding suicide risk and not limiting access to the means to realise it are fundamental to saving lives (REGISTRED NURSES' ASSOCIATION OF ONTARIO - RNAO, 2009; ENA, 2012; MENON, 2013; YIP et. aL, 2012). Approximately 90 per cent of people who died by suicide had at least one contact with a health professional in the three months prior to their death. This data points to the importance of these contacts being considered opportunities for suicide prevention (DE LEO et. aL, 2013).

The risk of suicide represents a critical situation marked by the client's fragility and instability. An evidence-based, rapid, humanised and effective approach can be decisive for the patient's prognosis.

There is no universally accepted set of procedures on how to deal with a suicidal or potentially suicidal individual. However, there are national and international guidelines on recommended care for clients with suicidal behaviour (RNAO, 2009; ENA, 2012; BRASIL, 2006).

Recommendations related to caring for the individual include: carrying out a comprehensive assessment, providing support, mobilising resources, working on the client's ambivalence and problem-solving, promoting protective factors and well-being and encouraging the reduction of feelings of shame, guilt and stigma (RNAO, 2009; ENA, 2012; BRASIL, 2006). The relevance of these actions must be considered, not only for the purpose of preventing the death of the individual, but also for the production of subjectivity, the identification of reasons to live and the reconstruction of meanings about the self and life.

Comprehensive care for individuals with suicidal behaviour must become a life-enhancing mechanism capable of giving new meaning to all the processes in the individual's life (KANTORSKI et al, 2000).

The World Health Organisation has launched a number of recommendations related to collective health, which include reducing the availability of and access to the means to commit suicide, improving health services, diagnostic procedures and treatment, strengthening social support, public education, adequacy of reporting of suicides and suicide attempts, training for individuals and professionals (WHO, 2004; WHO, 2005).

In addition, the WHO recommends research into suicide prevention and that greater attention be paid to health professionals in relation to their attitudes and taboos regarding suicide prevention and mental illness (WHO, 2004; WHO, 2005). These aspects are directly related to this study.

When it comes to suicide prevention, t's worth noting that the quality of care provided after a suicide attempt is particularly important, as these clients are at greater risk of making further attempts and carrying out the act (NEBHINANI et. aL, 2013), and these cases are initially treated in pre-hospital and hospital emergency services.

As a result of the increase in the number of cases of suicide and suicide attempts, these are increasingly present in the daily work of urgent and emergency care professionals (BERTOLOTE, MELLO-SANTOS, BOTEGA, 2010).

It should also be noted that nursing professionals in emergency services tend to be the first to have contact with patients after a suicice attempt or an episode of self-injury (CARMONA-NAVARRO; PICHARDO MARTÍNEZ, 2012), and nursing staff working in emergencies have frequent contact with clients after suicide attempts, playing a central role in the initial management of these cases (NEBHINANI et. aL, 2013; OSAFO et. aL, 2012).

In interventions aimed at suicide, health professionals face difficulties involving a lack of planning, inability to manage suicide risk and unavailability of resources (VANNOY et. aL, 2011).

Furthermore, health professionals tend to attribute widely varying meanings to suicidal behaviour, which are linked to attempts to get attention, solve or end suffering, an act of courage, a weak support network, a lack of prospects for the future and the presence of mental disorders (FREITAS; BORGES, 2014).

Care for suicidal clients can be influenced by a variety of factors, including attitudes towards suicide, professional training and the ability to assess suicide risk and plan care (DE LEO et. al. 2013; MENON, 2013; NEBHINANI et aL, 2013; OSAFO et aL, 2012; SRIVASTAVA, TIWARI, 2012).

The attitudes of healthcare professionals seem to have a significant positive or negative effect on patient care (FREITAS; BORGES, 2014), but knowledge about these issues is still scarce (ROTHES et al, 2014). Nursing professionals have a range of attitudes and beliefs that affect their professional activities and, in turn, the suicidal behaviour of patients (CARMONA-NAVARRO, 2012). Studies are therefore needed that incorporate an understanding of professionals' attitudes towards suicide (NEBHINANI et al, 2013; TALSETH, GILJE, 2007).

Measuring attitudes towards suicidal behaviour can help prevent suicide and reduce deaths by suicide (JOE, DANIEL, PATRICK, 2007).

Attitude can be defined as a response to a stimulus that involves cognitive, affective and behavioural components, extending to all aspects of intelligence and behaviour (ALTMANN, 2008). It is an inner disposition that affects decision-making or behaviour towards people, events or objectives.

Thus, attitude is not specifically behaviour, but propensity to action, ways or forms of approaching, reacting to or facing a situation or problem in a variety of circumstances. Some terms related to attitudes are opinions, points of view, lines of thought and postures; and some synonyms for attitude are perspective, position and way of thinking (ALTMANN, 2008).

According to some dictionaries, attitude can be defined as "a complex mental state involving beliefs and feelings and values and dispositions to act in certain ways" (DICTIONARY.COM, 2016), as well as "reaction or way of being towards people or objects" (FERREIRA, 2000).

The three characteristics most commonly found among definitions of attitudes are: conscious or unconscious mental states; value, belief or feeling; and predisposition towards a behaviour or action (ALTMANN, 2008). Thus, attitude is considered a psychological process that determines individual behaviour (ADJZEN, 1988).

Attitudes are commonly investigated by measuring them using validated quantitative instruments. There are various instruments for measuring attitudes related to suicidal behaviour, which differ in terms of form, content, method of application, target audience and analysis systems, each contributing to the understanding of specific aspects related to suicide (GHASEMI, SHAGHAGHI, ALLAHVERDIPOUR, 2015).

This study used the "Questionnaire of Attitudes to Suicidal Behaviour (QACS)", which was designed to be applied to health professionals, with the aim of verifying the attitudes of these individuals towards the behaviour in question (BOTEGA, 2005). This instrument makes it possible to investigate these attitudes in their cognitive, affective and behavioural components, i.e. in addition to attitudes, associated factors can be verified.

Studies show that emergency professionals generally have negative attitudes towards caring for suicidal patients (SUOMINEN, SUOKAS, LÕNNQVIST, 2007) and there is also resistance on the part of health professionals to attending to mental health patients (BERTOLOTE, MELLO-SANTOS, BOTEGA, 2010). Studies also reveal the existence of misconceptions about suicide among health teams, who tend to underestimate the risk of suicide or ignore the patient and fail to take advantage of opportunities to carry out prevention (CREPALDI, 2012; XIAOHUI et aL, 2015).

In the literature, the relationship between attitudes and factors such as gender, age, length of clinical experience and previous education is still unclear (KELLY, MACCARTHY, SAHM, 2014).

Understanding the attitudes attributed to suicide by nursing professionals can facilitate the understanding of experiences and behaviours related to suicidal behaviour.

Nursing care for these people must be based on scientific evidence, but it must also consider and value the uniqueness of the people being cared for and incorporate new ways of looking at and thinking about psychological suffering as a phenomenon of existence, without reproducing static and crystallised models, typical of exclusionary models such as the asylum (HECK et aL, 2012).

Understanding nursing professionals' attitudes towards suicide can contribute to actions aimed at improving care. In addition, studies relating to nursing professionals' attitudes towards suicide need to consider the variations that exist in different countries, cultures and times (NEBHINANI et. aL, 2013; TALSETH; GILJE, 2007). Carrying out high-quality research and sensitising teams are crucial components in promoting changes in the general population's attitudes towards suicide in developing countries (POREDDI et aL, 2016).

This study hypothesised that attitudes towards suicide would be associated with gender, age, health service (pre-hospital or hospital), training and professional category, specific training in suicide, training in mental health, length of time working as a nurse and experience working in a psychiatric or mental health service. In this way, the results of this study can help to plan academic training strategies, continuing education, supervision strategies and support for the team, thus contributing to the health of professionals and improving care.

CHAPTER 2

Objective

The aim of this study was to investigate attitudes towards suicide and associated factors among nursing professionals working in emergency departments.

CHAPTER 3

Method

3.1 Research design

The researcher is faced with a variety of methodological choices and these must be coherent with the research and enable the objectives to be achieved.

Quantitative research covers a broad spectrum and includes studies with data collection methods that use questionnaires to measure participants' attitudes (MEADOWS, 2003), as is the case in this study.

Quantitative research enables deductive reasoning, the formulation of hypotheses based on the systematisation of a problem and the choice of mechanisms capable of investigating it, taking into account the control and minimisation of possible biases, as well as maximising precision and validity, with results capable of being generalised (POLIT, BECK, HUNGLER, 2011). Considering all these characteristics and its suitability for achieving the objectives of this study, we opted for quantitative research.

This study used a quantitative, cross-sectional approach, as the variables were identified and determined at a point in time (HARTUNG, TOCHETTE, 2009; SOUSA, DRIESSNACK, MENDES, 2007).

3.2 Study sites

The research was carried out in two urgent and emergency care centres located in the interior of the state of São Paulo, Brazil.

A hospital complex for urgent and emergency care, belonging to a public university hospital that is primarily a tertiary care centre. This service consists of a Clinical Stabilisation Room for clinical problems, a Trauma Room for polytraumatised patients, a Sector for non-traumatic emergency care for less serious patients and a Psychiatry Sector.

The other place alluded to in this study is the Mobile Emergency Care Service (SAMU), which has Basic Life Support Units and Advanced Support Units, which carry out pre-hospital urgent and emergency care in the context in which it occurs. The service is requested via a free phone call to 192, which is used nationwide, and organised by the Regulation Centres. In the city where this study took place, healthcare is organised through a network of services, made up of five Districts located in the North, South, East, West and Central regions. SAMU has established its operational bases located in each of the Health Districts to offer basic and emergency care close to users' homes.

These services were chosen because they provide direct assistance to patients at risk of suicide or post-attempt.

3.3 Study participants

All nursing professionals who worked in the two urgent and emergency care centres where the study was carried out and who met the selection criteria were invited to take part in the study.

The population of nursing professionals (nurses, nursing assistants and technicians) at the study sites who reported having seen patients at risk of or attempting suicide were eligible to take part in the study. Professionals under the age of 18 or who were not actively working in the health institution surveyed during the data collection period were excluded.

According to information provided by the study sites, the nursing staff employed totalled 173 professionals, 27 of whom were nurses and 146 nursing assistants or technicians. Of these, seven professionals were excluded because they were on sick leave or on leave of absence, eight were excluded from the study because they reported not having seen any patients at risk of or attempting suicide and 12 people refused to take part. The participants in this study thus totalled 146 people.

3.4 Data Collection

Data collection took place between April and December 2015, following consent from the services and approval by the Research Ethics Committee under Protocol CAAE: 40072214.0.0000.5393 (Annex A).

Before data collection began, a brief presentation of the project was made to the directors of the emergency unit and the SAMU, explaining what would be done. The directors of nursing at the SAMU and the emergency unit were asked for a list of all the active employees in the services and the duty rosters, containing the days, times, full names and sectors of each professional. At the same time, a brief visit was made to the sectors where the data was collected. All this information favoured the planning of this collection.

Each participant received explanations about the nature of this research, its objective, the procedures that would be carried out, ethical aspects and voluntary participation. The average collection time with each participant was between 20 and 30 minutes.

The researcher used a private area, which did not jeopardise either the professional or the running of the service. The instruments were self-applied. We endeavoured to follow this sequence:

- The Free and Informed Consent Form (FICF) was read and completed. Two copies were signed, with one copy remaining with the participant and one with the researcher;

- The participant was asked to answer the sociodemographic questionnaire;

- Orientation on the QACS was carried out, following only the instructions contained in the instrument, which shows how to fill it in using examples. There was no discussion about where to tick the box, nor was there any induction on how to do it.

Nursing professionals who met the inclusion criteria individually filled in the data contained in the following instruments:

- Informed Consent Form (Appendix A);
- Sociodemographic questionnaire (Appendix B);
- Questionnaire on Attitudes to Suicidal Behaviour - QACS (Annex B).

3.4.1 Sociodemographic questionnaire (Appendix B):

A script was used to collect sociodemographic data, containing questions related to gender (female or male), service (Trauma Room, Clinical Stabilisation Room, Box, Psychiatry or SAMU), role (assistant, technician or nurse), age, training (technical/professional training, incomplete higher education, complete higher education, specialisation/residency, master's degree, doctorate), specific training in mental health, length of time working in nursing and in the ward of professional practice (years), experience in mental health or psychiatry services, and whether they had received specific training in suicide.

3.4.2 Questionnaire on Attitudes to Suicidal Behaviour - QACS (Annex B):

The Questionnaire of Attitudes to Suicidal Behaviour (QACS) is a Brazilian instrument, with an individual approach and self-application, developed by José Neury Botega and collaborators in 2005, specifically to measure the attitudes of nursing professionals to suicidal behaviour (BOTEGA et aL, 2005).

The instrument was developed due to the theoretical and practical limitations of the instruments available to measure attitudes. To develop the QACS, a literature review and focus groups with nursing professionals were first carried out to develop the statements that would make up the instrument. Initially, 54 statements related to attitudes were extracted. The relevance and appropriateness of the statements were assessed by specialists (they were reduced to 25 items) and submitted to a pilot test, which resulted in the elimination of four phrases, one for being poorly formulated and the other three for presenting low variation in responses (BOTEGA et aL, 2005; CAIS et aL, 2011).

Thus, 21 statements were selected. Each statement is followed by a ten-centimetre visual analogue scale (10 points) ranging from "strongly disagree" at one end to "strongly agree" at the other.

The scale's internal consistency was assessed by factor analysis, using maximum likelihood and Varimax orthogonal rotation. Three interpretable factors were extracted, together accounting for 43 per cent of the total variance (BOTEGA et al, 2005). Thus, in the original study, the items were grouped into three factors: 1- Feelings towards the patient; 2- Perception of professional capacity; and 3- Right to Suicide. Cronbach's *alpha* coefficient was calculated for each factor, and the results obtained were 0.7, 0.6 and 0.5 respectively. The score for each of the three factors created can vary between zero and 30 points.

It should be noted that the instrument does not have cut-off points for the scores, which categorise the results, and can be analysed using the three factors, as well as by analysing the 21 items in isolation. The author of the QACS questionnaire authorised its use in this study (Appendix C).

The following are the factors of the instrument, the items that make them up and how to interpret the results obtained:

1. Feelings towards the patient:

This factor includes the items:
5.*"Deep down, I prefer not to get too involved with patients who have attempted suicide'"*,
13.*"Deep down, sometimes it makes me angry, because so many people want to live... and that patient wants to die[1] '*; and
15. "We *feel powerless in the face of a person who wants to kill themselves[1] '-*, The higher the score on this factor, the greater the presence of such feelings.

2. Perception of professional capacity:

This factor shows the sum of the values obtained in the items:
1.*"I feel able to help a person who has tried to kill themselves"*;
10. *"I am professionally trained to deal with patients at risk of suicide"*; and

12. *"I feel insecure about caring for patients at risk of suicide"* (with inverted value).

A higher score can mean that professionals are more confident in dealing with individuals with suicidal behaviour.

3. *Right to Suicide:*

For this factor 3, the sum comes from the items:

3. *"Despite everything, I think that if a person wants to kill themselves, they have the right to do so."*

6. *"Life is a gift from God, and only he can take it away"* (with inverted value); and

16. *"Those who have God in their hearts won't try to kill themselves"* (inverted).

In terms of interpreting the values obtained in this analysis of factor 3, a higher score may represent a less "moralistic/judgemental" attitude.

The interviewees were asked to indicate only one point on each line that best reflected their opinions, feelings or reactions. All documents were collected after participation.

The score for each item on the QACS was taken from the point of intersection between the line available on the instrument and the line drawn by the study participant. The score was calculated in centimetres and the values were transferred to the database to one decimal place.

The time and place for the data collection were agreed with the participants, in agreement with the health service managers, so as not to jeopardise the activities carried out in their workplaces.

3.5 Analysing the data

After applying the Questionnaire of Attitudes towards Suicidal Behaviour (QACS) (BOTEGA et al, 2005), the data was structured in spreadsheet format in Microsoft Excel and then transferred to the Statistical Package for the Social Sciences (SPSS) software, version 19.0 and R GUI 3.0.1, avoiding possible errors in the analysis, consistency and veracity of the data obtained (PALLANT, 2010). Double-entering the data allowed for greater certainty in its veracity and the stability of the results, as there was a comparison of the data that was entered at two different times, one by the researcher and the other by the collaborators.

Measurement assigns numbers to the qualities of each object, designating their quantitative attributes, as long as rules are used to eliminate guesswork and ambiguity throughout the process of gathering and communicating information (POLIT, BECK, HUNGLER, 2011). The use of descriptive statistics for the variables studied allowed for distribution in percentages, mean with standard deviation and median.

The Kolmogorov-Smirnova and Shapiro-Wilk normality tests were applied, showing results of asymmetrical distribution, with positive and negative slopes. Therefore, all the variables (gender, age, specific training in mental health, experience of working in a psychiatric or mental health service, specific training in suicide, position - nurse, technician or nursing assistant -, length of time working in nursing and question 21 of the QACS) did not have normal distributions across the three factors analysed.

Sociodemographic variables (gender, mental health training, mental health experience, suicide training, hospital or pre-hospital service, role as nurse, technician or nursing assistant) were tested and associated with the QACS factors using the Mann-Witney test and standard deviation. The non-parametric Mann-Witney U test was used due to non-normal distribution. The minimum *alpha* level accepted in scientific research, which is 0.05 (p<0.05), was used in this study. It indicates that with a significance level *(alpha* or a) of 0.05 there would only be five null hypotheses being incorrectly rejected in every 100 samples, i.e. compared to the confidence intervals (CI) 0.05 would be equal to 95 per cent (POLIT, BECK, HUNGLER, 2011).

The results were validated using Spearman's correlation test, applied to question 21 "Have I ever been in situations that made me think about committing suicide" and "length of service". Pearson's correlation test, represented by *r,* is a measure of the degree of linear correlation between two numerical variables (VIEIRA, 2008). This test allows us to describe the direction and magnitude of a relationship between two variables and the ranges +1.00 (correlation

(perfect positive correlation), through (0.00) to - 1.00 (perfect negative correlation) (POLIT, BECK, HUNGLER, 2011).

3.6 Ethical aspects

Those responsible for the health services authorised the study, which was approved by the Research Ethics Committee (Protocol CAAE: 40072214.0.0000.5393).

The study followed the recommendations of Resolution 466/2012 on research involving human beings (BRASIL, 2012). The study participants were informed about the anonymity and confidentiality of their information and their freedom to stop taking part in the research if necessary, without any personal harm being caused. Participation was voluntary and not for profit. They were also informed about the aims of the study and that the data obtained would be used to prepare a scientific paper and possibly published.

After verbally consenting to take part in the research, the participants were asked to sign the Informed Consent Form (Appendix A).

CHAPTER 4

Results

Characterisation of the study participants

Table 1 shows the distribution of sociodemographic characteristics, professional experience and training of nursing professionals who worked in pre-hospital and hospital emergencies.

Table 1 - Sociodemographic characteristics, training and professional experience of the nursing professionals participating in the study (n=146). Ribeirão Preto, SP, Brazil, 2015-2016.

Variable description	n	%
Gender		
Male	30	20,5
Female	114	78,1
Missing	2	1,4
Age group (years)		
19-29	9	6,2
30-39	52	35,6
40-49	45	30,8
50-59	35	24,0
≥ 60	3	2,0
Missing	2	1,4
Time working in nursing (years)		
≤ 1 year	2	1,3
2-10	33	22,6
11-20	73	**50,0**
21 -30	29	19,9
≥31	9	6,2
Length of time working at the study site (years)		
≤ 1 year	27	18,5
>1 -10	59	40,4
11-20	48	32,9
≥21	12	8,2
Service		
Hospital	68	46,6
Pre-hospital	78	53,4
Function		
Nurse	28	19,2
Nursing Technician	55	37,7
Nursing assistant	63	43,1
Mental health training		
Yes	36	24,7
No	110	75,3
Experience in psychiatry or mental health		
Yes	36	247
No	110	75,3
Suicide training		
Yes	17	11,6
No	129	88,4

146 nursing professionals took part in the study. The age of the interviewees ranged from 25 to 63 years, with a mean of 43 years, and the majority of the professionals were under 50 years

of age (72.5%) at the time of data collection.

The length of time they had worked in nursing ranged from three months to 36 years, with an average of 16 years.

The majority of professionals were female (78.1%), worked in pre-hospital services (53.4%), had been working in nursing for more than 10 years (75.9%), were nursing technicians or assistants (80.9%), had no specific training in mental health (75.3%) or training in suicide (88.4%) and had no experience of working in mental health services (75.3%).

Nursing professionals' attitudes towards suicide

Table 2 shows the answers given by nursing professionals to the questions in the Questionnaire on attitudes towards suicidal behaviour.

Table 2 - Scores obtained by nursing professionals on the items in the Questionnaire on attitudes towards suicidal behaviour. Ribeirão Preto, São Paulo, 2015-2016.

Question	Range obtained	Median	Mean (SD)
Q1 I feel able to help someone who has tried to kill themselves;	0,00 -10,0	7,90	7,34 (2,75)
Q2 People who threaten usually don't kill themselves;	0,00 -10,0	0,40	3,56 (3,18)
Q3 Despite everything, I think that if a person wants to kill themselves, they have the right to do so;	0,00 -10,0	1,80	1,51 (3,00)
Q4 When faced with a suicide, I think: if someone had talked to them, they would have found another way;	0,00 -10,0	7,75	7,37 (2,69)
Q5 Basically, I prefer not to get too involved with patients who have attempted suicide;	0,00 -10,0	1,80	2,64 (3,00)
Q6 Life is a gift from God, and only he can take it away;	0,00 -10,0	9,90	8,71 (2,78)
Q7 I feel able to realise when a patient is at risk of killing themselves;	0,00 -10,0	6,05	5,97 (2,79)
Q8 People who kill themselves usually have a	0,00 -10,0	2,35	3,34 (3,40)

mental illness;			
Q9 I'm afraid to ask about ideas of suicide, and end up inducing the patient to do so;	0,00 -10,0	1,90	2,98 (3,29)
Q10 I am professionally trained to deal with patients at risk of suicide;	0,00 -10,0	4,90	5,22 (3,21)
Q11 It takes a certain amount of courage to kill yourself;	0,00 -10,0	8,10	7,13(3,39)
Q12 I feel insecure about caring for patients at risk of suicide;	0,00 -10,0	2,65	3,36 (3,34)
Q13 Deep down, sometimes it makes you angry, because so many people want to live... and that patient wants to die;	0,00 -10,0	2,70	3,73 (3,61)
Q14 If I suggest a psychiatric inter-consultation for a patient who has talked about killing himself, I think this will be well accepted by his treating doctor;	0,00 -10,0	7,00	6,49 (3,03)
Q15 We feel powerless in the face of someone who wants to kill themselves;	0,00 -10,0	4,65	4,74 (3,11)
Q16 Those who have God in their hearts won't try to kill themselves;	0,00 -10,0	4,70	5,00 (3,70)
Q17 In the case of patients who are suffering greatly from a physical illness, I find the idea of suicide more acceptable;	0,00 -10,0	0,60	1,85 (2,97)
Q18 When someone talks about ending their life, I try to take their mind off it;	0,00 -10,0	9,50	8,76 (2,05)
Q19 People who really want to kill themselves don't "try" to kill themselves;	0,00 -10,0	4,40	4,40 (3,78)
Q20 A hospitalised patient is unlikely to kill themselves without a strong motive;	0,00 -10,0	3,10	3,85 (3,41)
Q21 I've been in situations that made me think about committing suicide;	0,00-10,0	0,00	1,69 (3,40)

SD (Standard Deviation)

The minimum (0) and maximum (10) scores for each of the items in the questionnaire were obtained, which means that there were people who fully agreed and people who fully disagreed with each of the statements in the questionnaire.

The average score for the 21 questions was 4.38 points. The statement with the lowest median score was the question *"I've been through situations that made me think about committing suicide"* (0.00) and the question with the lowest mean score was *"Despite everything, I think that if a person wants to kill themselves, they have the right to do so"* (1.51). These scores indicate greater disagreement with the statements.

It should be noted that although question 21 had a low mean score (1.69) and median (0.00), the range obtained on this question was from 0 to 10, with nine participants fully agreeing with this statement.

The statement with the highest median score was *"Life is a gift from God, and only He can take it away"* (9.90) and the highest mean score was *"When a person talks about ending their life, I try to get it out of their head"* (8.76). These were the statements with which the interviewees expressed the most agreement.

Table 3 shows the results obtained in the QACS factors: 1- Feelings towards the patient; 2- Perception of professional capacity; and 3- Right to Suicide. The score for each factor can vary from zero to 30 points.

Table 3 - Scores obtained by nursing professionals (N=146) in the factors of the Questionnaire of Attitudes towards Suicidal Behaviour (QACS). Ribeirão Preto, SP, Brazil, 2016.

Factor	Range obtained	Median	Mean (SD)
1-. Negative feelings towards the patient	0,0-30,0	10,60	11,44 (6,58)
2- Perception of professional capacity	0,0-30,0	19,70	18,78 (7,02)
3- Right to Suicide	0,0-30,0	8,05	8,44 (6,37)

SD (Standard Deviation)

Compared to the other factors, factor 3 had the lowest median (8.05) and mean (8.44) values, while factor 2 had the highest median (19.70) and mean (18.78) values.

Table 4 shows the comparisons between the means obtained in the QACS, according to the variables related to sociodemographic characteristics and those related to professional training and experience.

Table 4 - Sociodemographic characteristics, training and professional experience of nursing professionals according to the scores obtained in the factors of the Questionnaire of Attitudes towards Suicidal Behaviour (QACS) (n=146). Ribeirão Preto, SP, Brazil, 2016.

Variable	Factor 1		Factor 2		Factor3	
	Mean (SD)	P-value	Mean (SD)	P-value	Mean (SD)	P-value
Sex		0,80		0,24		0,34
Female	11,43 (6,90)		18,43 (7,01)		8,13(6,15)	
Male	11,47 (5,41)		20,03 (7,02)		9,52 (7,09)	
Mental Health Training		0,28		**0,00**		0,14
Yes	10,42 (6,89)		24,23(4,91)		10,40 (7,10)	
No	11,51 (6,59)		18,42 (7,00)		8,31 (6,33)	
Experience in Mental Health		**0,00**		0,15		**0,01**
Yes	8,80 (5,15)		20,03 (5,88)		10,22 (6,64)	
No	12,37 (6,80)		18,35 (7,36)		7,82 (6,19)	
Suicide counselling		0,43		**0,00**		0,76
Yes	11,07 (6,98)		24,34 (3,68)		7,78 (7,51)	
No	11,49 (6,36)		18,06 (7,04)		8,53 (6,24)	
Function		0,37		0,55		**0,00**
Nurse	11,30 (6,76)		18,02 (8,54)		12,16(6,18)	
Auxiliary/ Technical	11,48 (6,57)		18,97(6,64)		7,56 (6,12)	
Service		0,87		**0,01**		0,27
Hospital	10,66 (5,87)		20,09 (6,80)		8,58 (5,97)	
Pre-hospital	12,12 (7,12)		17,66 (7,06)		8,32 (6,74)	

Test used: Mann-Witney; SD (Standard Deviation)

In factor 1, which indicates more negative attitudes towards suicide, people with experience of having worked in a mental health service scored higher (p=0.00).

Higher scores on factor 2, which reveal a greater perception of professional capacity, were present among professionals with specific training in mental health (p=0.00), among those who had already received specific training related to suicide (p=0.00) and among those who worked in hospital services (p=0.01).

With regard to factor 3, people with experience in mental health services (p=0.01) and nurses scored higher (less moralistic/judgemental attitude) than technicians and assistants (p=0.00). There was no significant difference between men and women with regard to the factors.

Spearman's correlation test was applied to test correlations between QACS factors and the continuous numerical variables length of experience and the score on question 21. The results of the test are shown in Table 5.

Table 5 - Scores obtained by nursing professionals in the factors of the Questionnaire of Attitudes towards Suicidal Behaviour (QACS) according to the score obtained in question 21 of the QACS and length of professional experience (n=146). Ribeirão Preto, SP, Brazil, 2016.

Domain		Time Experience	Q21
Factor 1	Spearman coefficient*	-0,04	0,11
	p-value	0,96	0,16
	n	146	145
Factor 2	Spearman coefficient*	0,03	-0,06
	p-value	0,66	0,45
	n	146	145
Factor 3	Spearman coefficient*	0,02	0,03
	p-value	0,81	0,68
	n	146	145

There was no correlation between the QACS factors and the variables length of experience and the score on question 21. However, there was a weak negative correlation (r= -0.302) between factors 1 and 2 (p=0.00), meaning that people with a higher perception of professional capacity had less negative attitudes towards suicidal behaviour.

CHAPTER 5

Discussion

According to the World Health Organsation, more than 450 million people have some kind of mental disorder or psychological problem (WHO, 2001). Therefore, at some point, professionals working in different healthcare contexts will come into contact with patients with mental health issues. These include psychiatric emergencies.

Psychiatric emergencies are alterations of a psychiatric nature in which changes in the mental state result in a current and significant risk cf death or serious injury to the patient or third parties (QUEVEDO, SCHMITT, KAPCZINSKI, 2008).

These conditions are prevalent and challenging. It is estimated that approximately 53 million psychiatric emergencies occurred in the United States between 1992 and 2001 (LARKIN, SMITH, BEAUTRAIS, 2008). Between 2001 and 2011 in the United States, psychiatric emergencies increased from 4.4% to 7.2% of total emergency department attendances, which is equivalent to 55,000 more attendances each year during this period (SIMON, SCHOENDORF, 2014).

Urgent and emergency care services play an essential role in dealing with psychiatric crises (BRASIL, 2002). In Brazil, the main care facilities for acute cases are the Psychosocial Care Centres (CAPS), general and emergency psychiatric hospitals and the Mobile Emergency Care Service (SAMU) (BRASIL, 2001).

It is important that emergency care services are easily accessible and prepared to deal with psychiatric emergencies, as they can play an important role in preventing illnesses (ANSSEAU, et aL, 2004; FULBROOK, LAWRENCE, 2015). In many cases, these services are a gateway to mental health services (DOWNEY, ZUN, BURKE, 2012).

Emergency services are characterised by high turnover, a variety of clinical cases, complexity and excessive demand, which can make them unattractive to health professionals (DEL-BEN, TENG, 2010).

The field of urgencies and emergencies is challenging and requires highly trained professionals (ANTAI-OTONG, 2016). However, nurses' academic training often does not focus on aspects related to mental health and psychatric emergencies (GIRADE, CRUZ, STEFANELLI, 2006). In this context, more humanised approaches, such as attentive listening and a helping relationship, are underused, and when they do occur, they are fraught with difficulties related to the incorporation of the biomedical model into clinical care, excessive use of medication and mechanical restraint (SANTOS, COIMBRA, RIBEIRO, 2011).

Psychiatric emergencies include suicide attempts and suicidal behaviour as a whole. Suicide is a major public health problem that can be prevented. The World Health Organisation has set itself the goal of achieving at least a 10% reduction in the number of suicides worldwide by 2020 (WHO, 2014). To achieve this, it is necessary to invest in prevention strategies.

Previous suicide attempts are the main risk factor for future suicide (OWENS, HORROCKS, HOUSE, 2002), and the person's risk of committing suicide increases according to the number of attempts and is also linked to the length of time between these attempts (BERTOLOTE, MELLO-SANTOS, BOTEGA, 2010; QUEVEDO, SCHMITT, KAPCZINSKI, 2008; VIDAL, GONTIJO, 2013). This clientele is at greater risk of making further attempts and committing suicide and deserves special attention in terms of prevention (WHO, 2006).

Thus, the care provided to people who have attempted suicide in emergency services can be decisive for the prognosis of these individuals, as qualified assessment and intervention regarding suicidal risk and limited access to the means to realise it are fundamental to saving lives (RNAO, 2009; ENA, 2012; MENON, 2013; YIP et aL, 2012). However, when caring for people with suicidal behaviour, health professionals face difficulties involving lack of planning, inability to manage suicide risk and unavailability of resources (VANNOY et aL, 2011).

As a result of the increase in the number of cases of suicide and suicide attempts, these are increasingly present in the daily work of emergency professionals (BERTOLOTE et al, 2010). It is noteworthy that nursing professionals in emergency services tend to be the first to have contact with patients after a suicide attempt or an episode of self-injury (CARMONA-NAVARRO, PICHARDO MARTÍNEZ, 2012), have frequent contact with clients after suicide attempts and play a central role in the initial management of these cases (OSAFO et. al., 2012; NEBHINANI et. al., 2013).

Caring for suicidal clients can be influenced by various factors, including the attitudes of nursing professionals (DE LEO et al., 2013; NEBHINANI et al., 2013; SRIVASTAVA et al., 2012; OSAFO et al., 2012; MENON, 2013), which were investigated in this study.

Attitudes towards suicide in this study were associated with experience of working in a mental health service, place of work, role held, specific training in mental health and specific training related to suicide. These results could subsidise actions aimed at improving care.

A recent literature review found that nurses from various health sectors play a central role in caring for patients at risk of suicide, and that negative attitudes towards this behaviour are common among these professionals, indicating that educating these professionals through reflective and interactive components can provide positive changes in attitudes towards suicide. Furthermore, it emphasises that improving care requires adequate training, resources and time to develop appropriate patient care techniques (KARMAN et al., 2015).

The results of this study revealed that nursing professionals have little specific educational exposure to the subject of suicide. However, education related to suicide prevention offered to health professionals can improve these individuals' attitudes towards suicide avoidance, clarity of their role, confidence and more preventive attitudes towards suicide (RAMBERG, LUCCA, HADLACZKY, 2016). In this sense, it is important to question why there is little educational exposure to such a relevant topic on the national and world stage.

This problem does not seem to be peculiar to the context studied. A study carried out in China found that in hospital urgent and emergency care services, training is often geared towards demands unrelated to mental health and the barriers to preparing teams to deal with psychiatric emergencies are the complexity of the emergency care process, prejudice, lack of information about psychiatric emergencies and the possibility of suicide prevention (XIAOHIU et aL, 2015).

In this study, the relationship between training and attitudes proved to be complex. Specific training in suicide or mental health was associated with a greater perception of professional capacity, but was not associated with less condemnatory and negative attitudes. On the other hand, nurses (professionals with higher education) had a less moralistic/judgemental attitude compared to technicians and auxiliaries. These results point to the importance of educational strategies that incorporate attitudinal knowledge (and not just cognitive and procedural knowledge) to promote more positive, empathetic and welcoming attitudes towards people at risk of suicide.

Another result found in this study was that professionals who perceived themselves to be better prepared for suicide-related care had fewer negative attitudes. The literature shows that the acquisition of knowledge seems to be associated with more positive attitudes among professionals (MCCARTHY, GIJBELS, 2010). In addition, reflective and interactive education can contribute to reducing negative attitudes, as well as improving the way nurses work when caring for people with suicidal behaviour (KARMAN et al., 2015).

Nurses had less condemnatory attitudes than nursing assistants and technicians. In this respect, studies state that the training of nursing assistants has significant deficits (OESEBURG, HILBERTS, ROODBOL, 2015) and that nurses with more training or postgraduate degrees have more positive attitudes towards suicidal behaviour (MCCARTHY, GIJBELS, 2010; WHEATLEY, AUSTIN-PAYNE, 2009).

In general, the literature indicates that professional training is often insufficient to meet the demands of caring for patients who self-injure and recommends support groups and clinical supervision that can improve the care offered by nursing professionals (WHEATLEY, AUSTIN-

PAYNE, 2009). Continuing education offered to professionals within their work routine and contractual workload increases adherence to educational activities (CICONET, MARQUES, LIMA, 2008).

The literature shows that professionals with training in mental health have more positive attitudes towards suicide (SRIVASTAVA, TIWARI, 2012). However, in this study, specific training in mental health was only associated with a greater perception of professional capacity, which may favour the professional's sense of security in dealing with people at risk of suicide, but does not guarantee a more empathetic, less condemnatory and negative attitude.

Some studies have shown that preparing nurses on the subject of suicide through short workshops, self-directed studies or short courses favours safer behaviour and more positive attitudes towards suicide (PATTERSON, WHITTINGTON, BOGG, 2007; DICKINSON, WRIGHT, HARRISON, 2009). However, another study found no relationship between prior preparation about suicide and better attitudes (MCCARTHY, GIJBELS, 2010). In addition, mental health professionals consider that, in order to provide better care, more extensive education is needed (NORHEIM et aL, 2016).

Continuing education often involves qualifying people who already have strongly established technical knowledge, values and attitudes. In this sense, promoting changes in knowledge, skills and attitudes can be a challenge. Spaces for reflection are essential, as they are in continuing education, favouring the redefinition of practices, work, conduct and new strategies (CICONET, MARQUES, LIMA, 2008). Nurse education can also be provided by the application of protocols that guide their behaviour and contribute to the assessment of suicide risks and protective factors (ANTAI-OTONG, 2016).

The teaching-learning process must take into account the experiences of individuals and their professional and personal backgrounds, and not just the transfer of technical content, standards and guidelines, in order to enable important exchanges between subjects, the integration of knowledge, the sharing of experiences and feelings (ZANI, NOGUEIRA, 2006).

In this study, professionals who had previous experience of working in a mental health service (p=0.00) had more negative attitudes towards the patient, but they also had less condemnatory attitudes. In the literature, the relationship between clinical experience and attitudes towards suicide is not sufficiently clear (KELLY, MCCARTHY, SAHM, 2014).

There are varying results among studies in this regard, as no correlation has been identified between professional experience and attitudes (WHEATLEY, AUSTIN-PAYNE, 2009), but there are also indications that attitudes become more negative with the passage of time working with suicidal patients (DICKINSON, WRIGHT, HARRISON, 2009).

Studies show that nursing professionals have more negative attitudes towards people with suicidal behaviour or self-harm than other patients (SAUNDERS et aL, 2012; CARMONA-NAVARRO, PICHARDO- MARTÍNEZ, 2012). Negative attitudes towards suicidal behaviour are linked to the judgement of unpreparedness (XIAOHUI et. aL, 2015), and can reinforce the stigma experienced by people who have attempted suicide and their family members (PINTO-FOLTZ, LOGSDON, 2009; KARMAN et aL, 2015), as well as encouraging discrimination and hindering care for people who attempt suicide (SAUNDERS, 2012).

Studies show that the experience of completed suicide generates emotional and behavioural reactions such as disbelief, isolation, fear, sadness, anger, impotence, frustration, guilt, feelings of inadequacy and embarrassment, as well as insecurity, making it an important psychological experience for healthcare professionals (SCOCCO et al, 2012; FAIRMAN et al, 2014). Negative attitudes towards suicidal behaviour can be characterised by anger, detachment and helplessness (BOTEGA et aL, 2005), which are identified among the reactions to a patient's suicide. Thus, there is a possibility that traumatic experiences of death by suicide can lead to negative attitudes if they are not properly dealt with.

These experiences of patient deaths by suicide can interfere with the mental health and clinical practice of professionals (TALSETH, GILJE, 2007), who are the first to have contact with suicidal patients or episodes of self-harm (CARMONA-NAVARRO, PICHARDO MARTÍNEZ, 2012), as well as having a central role in this care (KARMAN et al, 2015).

Emergency professionals are regularly exposed to traumatic experiences and are particularly susceptible to secondary traumatic stress, cumulative burnout and a state of physical and mental exhaustion (COCKER, JOSS, 2016). In addition, emergency services are highly demanding and present significant occupational risks, which can lead to emotional and physical damage and a high workload for professionals (REUTER, CAMBA, 2017).

Suicide can be a traumatic incident for society and the family, and often there are no bereavement programmes, and when there are, their effectiveness is questionable. Social and health professional support for the families of patients who have committed suicide is essential, as they are vulnerable, stigmatised and isolated, factors that favour the acquisition of depression (SPINO et aL, 2016). However, it should be borne in mind that professionals also need support in coping with situations related to suicide.

Preparing professionals to manage suicide is not limited to training, as professionals are also emotionally affected when providing care and can experience feelings of professional failure, reduced self-esteem, questioning of their own professional skills and competences (TALSETH, GILJE, 2007). The training and development of emotional competences enables nursing professionals to provide better care for suicidal people and to reduce negative attitudes towards suicidal behaviour (CARMONA-NAVARRO, PICHARDO-MARTÍNEZ, 2012).

Another element that may be associated with attitudes towards suicide is the professional environment. A previous study found that nurses who worked in mental health or small hospitals had more positive attitudes than those who worked in large hospitals (PATTERSON, WHITTINGTON, BOGG, 2007).

In this study, professionals in the pre-hospital service felt less prepared to deal with suicide than people in the hospital service. This may be related to the exposure of professionals to more challenging situations in the pre-hospital context. Pre-hospital services can be a highly demanding field in terms of providing treatment, care and transport, and professionals often feel inadequate in this system (REUTER, CAMBA, 2017).

In this study, in each of the statements in the questionnaire there was an indication of agreement and complete disagreement, i.e. markings in the space between the ends of the question. This shows that opinions and attitudes towards suicide were varied or divergent, which can make team cohesion difficult in some situations. It is therefore worth highlighting the importance of applying interventions to these teams that favour continuing education, team discussions, clinical supervision and that can foster a cohesive approach.

In general, the scores for the individual questions revealed a high level of disagreement with the person's right to decide on suicide. This attitude was also observed among general practitioners and emergency doctors (XIAOHIU et al, 2015). The idea that suicide is reprehensible and reprehensible can favour moralistic attitudes and more prescriptive approaches (OSAFO ET aL, 2012). Although it is not desirable for suicide to be an acceptable option, it is important to beware of extremist, judgemental or unempathetic attitudes, as empathy and the therapeutic bond are necessary for the implementation of various care actions recommended in the management of suicide (ENA, 2012; MENON, 2013; RNAO, 2009).

There was no relationship between gender and attitudes towards suicidal behaviour, corroborating the results of other studies, as the existence of an association between gender and such attitudes is inconclusive in scientific literature (MCCARTHY, GIJBELS, 2010; KELLY, MCCARTHY, SAHM, 2014; SANTOS, COIMBRA, RIBEIRO, 2014; KARMAN ET aL, 2015).

No association was found between age and attitudes towards suicide. In this regard, a study in Ireland found that older nurses in urgent and emergency departments had more positive attitudes towards suicidal behaviour than younger nurses (CONLON, O'TUATHAIL, 2012). Another study found that the most positive attitudes were concentrated among nurses aged between 41 and 50 (MCCARTHY, GIJBELS, 2010).

Length of service in nursing was also not associated with attitudes towards suicidal behaviour. There is evidence that, in urgent and emergency care, with years of service, professionals' attitudes become more positive, but after a few years, they tend to become negative (MCCARTHY, GIJBELS, 2010).

It is also noteworthy that 6 per cent of the interviewees fully agreed with the expression "I have been in situations that have made me think about committing suicide". Thoughts and ideation are suicidal behaviours that deserve special attention to prevent the risk of suicide from progressing. It is therefore important to systematically assess the mental health of healthcare professionals, track the risk of suicide in this population and advance research and implementation of support interventions.

The occupational suffering experienced by professionals who work in emergencies generates feelings of impotence and flight in the face of pain (GARCIA et al., 2012). The proximity to death, especially in urgent and emergency care centres, is stressful for health professionals, especially nursing staff (GARCIA et al., 2012). In addition, the way in which individuals organise their work can lead to some degree of suffering (DEJOURS, 2015).

The identification of suffering and dissatisfaction among these professionals, the management of suffering and resources are fundamental to the psychological balance and mental health of these professionals (DEJOURS, 2015; GARCIA et al., 2016) and can even have an impact on the quality of care.

CHAPTER 6

Final considerations

The aim of this study was to investigate attitudes towards suicide and associated factors among nursing professionals working in emergency departments. To this end, the Attitudes to Suicidal Behaviour Questionnaire and a sociodemographic script were used to help achieve the proposed objectives.

It was found that nursing professionals had little educational exposure to suicide, but professionals who perceived themselves to be better prepared for suicide-related care had fewer negative attitudes.

The relationship between training and attitudes proved to be complex. Specific training in mental health or suicide was associated with a greater perception of professional capacity, but not with less negative or condemnatory attitudes. On the other hand, nurses (professionals with higher education) had a less moralistic/judgmental attitude compared to technicians and auxiliaries.

In this study, people with previous experience of working in a mental health service had more negative attitudes towards the patient, but they also had less condemnatory attitudes. Workplace was also associated with attitudes, with professionals in the pre-hospital service feeling less prepared to handle suicide than those in the hospital service. There was no association between attitudes towards suicidal behaviour and gender, age or length of time working in nursing.

It emerged that professionals have varied and sometimes divergent attitudes towards suicide, as there were responses indicating agreement and complete disagreement with each of the statements in the questionnaire used. In addition, in general, the scores for the individual questions showed a high level of disagreement with the right of the person to decide on suicide.

It is also noteworthy that 6 per cent of the interviewees reported having had suicidal thoughts, as they fully agreed with the expression *"I've been in situations that have made me think about committing suicide"*.

Based on the results obtained in this study and contributions from the scientific literature on the subject, corroborated with aspects found in the literature, here are some suggestions that can contribute to future studies, educational interventions and the improvement of professional practice:

- To investigate the reasons why there is little educational exposure to suicide, despite the relevance of this problem on the national and world stage;
- To assess the effectiveness, applicability and adherence of professionals to different educational strategies related to suicidal behaviour.

- Incorporate attitudinal knowledge and the development of emotional competences into educational strategies;
- Improving the approach to suicide in undergraduate and technical courses;
- Offering support, clinical supervision and continuing education on suicide;
- Encourage self-assessment and reflection on the perception of professional capacity and improvement strategies among emergency room nursing professionals;
- Encouraging self-knowledge and better management of stress and anxiety;
- We suggest that services provide moments for discussion, reflection and exchange of experiences that can favour the integration of knowledge, team cohesion, redefinition of practices and new care strategies;
- Use and evaluate protocols that guide the practice of nursing professionals;
- To assess the mental health of nursing professionals who work in urgencies and emergencies;

- To investigate the relationship between attitudes towards suicidal behaviour and traumatic experiences of death by suicide, professional environment, experience and length of time working in nursing, since these relationships are insufficiently clarified in the literature;
- To investigate the attitudes of nursing professionals towards suicidal behaviour in other contexts and using different methodological approaches.

The suggestions mentioned here were based on the analysis of the data from this study and supported by recommendations identified in the literature, and it is important to emphasise that the aforementioned interventions merit further investigation.

This study has some limitations, such as: cross-sectional design, the fact that it covers the population in specific contexts and the use of non-parametric tests, justified by the abnormality of the data distribution. Despite these limitations, this study is a pioneer in the investigation of factors associated with attitudes towards suicide among nursing professionals who work in emergencies in the Brazilian hospital and pre-hospital context.

This study allowed us to deepen our knowledge of suicide, which is a phenomenon present in the history of humanity, which has a significant global impact, is part of the daily life of health professionals, but which is still little addressed in society and has important gaps in the scientific literature.

Suicidal behaviour and clinical nursing practice are closely related, especially in the area of emergencies and urgencies. Suicidal risk represents a critical situation characterised by the client's fragility and instability. An evidence-based, rapid, humanised and effective approach can be decisive for the patient's prognosis. To achieve this, professionals need to be prepared and supported.

Given the importance of the topic of suicide and the path that can still be travelled in the field of research and professional practice, it is hoped that this work will be fertile and inspiring for other researchers, professionals, educators and managers.

REFERENCES

AJZEN, I. **Attitudes, personality and behaviour.** Milton Keynes: Open University Press, 1988.

ALTMANN, T. Attitude: a concept analysis. **Nursing Forum,** Sacramento, v. 43, n. 3, p. 144-150, 2008.

ANSSEAU, M.; DIERICK, M.; BUNTINKX, F.; SMEDT, J.; VAN DEN HAUTE, M.; VANDER MIJNSBRUGGE, D. High prevalence of mental disorders in primary care. **Journal of Affective Disorders,** Amsterdam, v. 78, n. 1, p. 49-55, 2004.

ANTAI-OTONG, D. What every ED nurse should know about suicide risk assessment. **Journal of Emergency Nursing,** St. Louis, v. 42, n. 3, p. 199- 200, 2016.

BERG, J. E. Which suicides increase during the economic crisis? A commentary and a proposal. **Journal of Public Health and Epidemiology,** Delta, v. 8, n. 5, p. 82-86, 2016.

BERTOLOTE, J. M.; MELLO-SANTOS, C.; BOTEGA, N. J. Detection of suicide risk in psychiatric emergency services. **Revista Brasileira de Psiquiatria,** São Paulo, v. 32, p. 87-95, 2010. Supplement 2.

BOTEGA, J. N. Suicidal behaviour: epidemiology. **Psicologia USP,** São Paulo, v. 25, n. 3, p. 231-236, 2014.

BOTEGA, N. J.; MARÍN-LEÓN, L.; OLIVEIRA, H. B.; BARROS, M. B.; SILVA, V. F.; DALGALARRONDO, P. Prevalence of suicide ideation, plans and attempts: a population-based survey in Campinas/SP. **Cadernos de Saúde Pública,** São Paulo, v. 25, n. 12, p. 2632-2638, 2009.

BOTEGA, N. J.; REGINATO, D. G.; SILVA, S. V.; CAIS, C. F. S.; RAPELI, C. B.; MAURO, M. L. F.; CECCONI, J. P.; STEFANELLO, S. Nursing personnel attitudes towards suicide: the development of a measure scale. **Revista Brasileira de Psiquiatria,** São Paulo, v. 27, n. 4, p. 315-318, 2005.

BRAZIL. Ministry of Health. **Law No. 10.216, of 6th April 2001.** Provides for the protection and rights of people with mental disorders and redirects the mental health care model. 2001. Available at: <http://www.planalto.gov.br/ccivil_03/leis/LEIS_2001/L10216.htm>. Accessed on: 30 October 2016.

BRAZIL. Ministry of Health. **Ordinance 2048/GM, of 5th November 2002.** Provides for the operation of Urgency and Emergency Services. Brasília: Ministry of Health, 2002.

BRAZIL. Ministry of Health. **Ordinance No. 1.876, of 14 August 2006.** Establishes National Guidelines for Suicide Prevention, to be implemented in all federal units, respecting the competences of the three spheres of management. 2006. Available at: <http://bvsms.saude.gov.br/bvs/saudelegis/gm/2006/prt1876_14_08_ 2006.html>. Accessed on: 30 May 2016.

BRAZIL. Ministry of Health. National Health Council. **Resolution No. 466/2012.** On research involving human beings. 2012. Available at: <http://conselho.saude.gov.br/resolucoes/2012/Reso466. pdf>. Accessed on: 10 October 2016.

CAIS, C. F. S.; SILVEIRA, I. U.; STEFANELLO, S.; BOTEGA, N. J. Suicide prevention training for professionals in the public health network in a large Brazilian city. **Archives of Suicide Research,** London, v. 15, n. 4, p. 384-389, 2011.

CARMONA-NAVARRO, M. C.; PICHARDC-MARTÍNEZ, M. C. Attitudes of nursing professionals towards suicidal behaviour: influence of emotional intelligence. **Revista Latino-Americana de Enfermagem,** São Paulo, v. 20, n. 6, p. 1161-1168, 2012.

CASSORLA, R. M. S. Suicide and human self-destruction. In: WERLANG, B. G.; BOTEGA, N. J. **Comportamento suicida.** Porto Alegre: Artmed, 2004.

CICONET, R. M.; MARQUES, G. Q.; LIMA, M. A. D. S. In-service education for health professionals in the Mobile Emergency Care Service (SAMU): An experience report from Porto Alegre-RS. **Interface,** Porto Alegre, v. 12, n. 26, p. 742-748, 2008.

CONLON, M.; O'TUATHAIL, C. Measuring emergency department nurses' attitudes towards deliberate self-harm using the self-harm antipathy scale. **International Emergency Nursing,** Oxford, v. 20, n. 1, p. 3-13, 2012.
COCKER, F.; JOSS, N. Compassion fatigue among healthcare, emergency and community Service workers: a systematic review. **International Journal of Environmental Research and Public Health,** Basel, v. 13, n. 618, p. 2-18, 2016.

CREPALDI, M. A. Preface. In: MALISKA, M. E.; WALLAUER. A. **Suicide:** a challenge for health professionals. Florianópolis: Pandion, 2012.

DEJOURS, C. **The madness of work:** a study of the psychopathology of labour. 6. ed. São Paulo: Cortez-Oboré, 2015.

DEL-BEN, C. M.; TENG, C. T. Psychiatric emergencies: challenges and vicissitudes. **Revista Brasileira de Psiquiatria,** São Paulo, v. 32, n. 2, p. 567-568, 2010.

DE LEO, D.; BURGIS, S.; BERTOLOTE, J. M.; KERKHOT, A. J.; BILLE-BRAHE, U. Definitions of suicidal behaviour. Lessons learnt from the WHO/HEN Multicentre Study. **Crisis,** Porto, v. 27, n. 1, p. 4-15, 2006.

DE LEO, D.; DRAPER, B. M.; SNOWDON, J.; KOLVES, K. Contacts with health professionals before suicide: missed opportunities for prevention? **Comprehensive Psychiatry,** New York, v. 54, n. 7, p. 1117-1123, 2013.

DICTIONARY.COM. Leraning somenthing every day. **Attitude.** 2015. Available at: <http://www.dictionary.com/browse/attitude?s=t>. Accessed on: 14 May 2016.

DICKINSON, T.; WRIGHT, K. M.; HARRISON, J. The attitudes of nursing staff in secure environments to young people who self-harm. **Journal of Psychiatric and Mental Health Nursing,** Oxford, v. 16, n. 10, p. 947-951,2009.

DOWNEY, L. A.; ZUN, L. S.; BURKE, T. Undiagnosed mental illness in the emergency department. **Journal of Emergency Medicine,** New York, v. 43, n. 1, p. 876-882, 2012.

DURKHEIN, E. **Suicide.** A sociological study. Rio de Janeiro: Zohar, 1982.

EMERGENCY NURSES ASSOCIATION (ENA). **Clinical practice guideline:** suicide risk assessment. Full version. ENA, 2012.
FAIRMAN, M. D. N.; THOMAS, L. L. P. M.; WHITMORE, S.; MEIER, E. A.; IRWIN, S. A. What did I miss? A qualitative assessment of impact of patient suicide on hospice staff. **Journal of Palliative Medicine,** Larchmont, v. 17, n. 10, p. 1-4, 2014.

FERREIRA, A. B. H. **Miniaurélio século XXI escolar.** Rio de Janeiro: Nova Fronteira, 2000.

FREITAS, A. P. A.; BORGES, L. M. Suicide attempts and health professionals: possible meanings. **Estudos e Pesquisas em Psicologia,** Rio de Janeiro, v. 14, n. 2, p. 560-577, 2014.

FULBROOK, P.; LAWRENCE, P. Survey of an Australian general emergency department: estimated prevalence of mental health disorders. **Journal of Psychiatric and Mental Health Nursing,** Boston, v. 22, n. 1, p. 30-38, 2015.

GARCIA, A. B.; DELLAROZA, M. S. G.; HADDAD, M. C. F. L. PACHEMSHY, L. R. Pleasure in the work of nursing technicians in the emergency department of a public university hospital. **Revista Gaúcha de Enfermagem,** Porto Alegre, v. 33, n. 2, p. 153-159, 2012.

GARCIA, A. B.; HADDAD, M. C. F. L.; DELLAROZA, M. S. G.; ROCHA, F. L. R.; PISSINATI, P. S. C. Strategies used by nursing technicians to cope with occupational distress in an emergency room. **Revista da Rede de Enfermagem do Nordeste,** Fortaleza, v. 17, n. 2, p. 285-292, 2016.

GIRADE, M. G.; CRUZ, M N. T.; STEFANELLI, M. C. Continuing education in psychiatric nursing: reflection on concepts. **Revista da Escola de Enfermagem,** São Paulo, v. 40, n. 1, p. 105-110, 2006.

GHASEMI, P.; SHAGHAGHI, A.; ALLAHVERDIPOUR, H. Measurement scales of suicidal ideation and attitudes: a systematic review article. **Health Promotion Perspective,** Tabriz, v. 5, n. 3, p. 156-168, 2015.

GOUDA, M. R. N., RAO, S. M. Factors Related to Attempted Suicide in Davanagere. **Indian Journal of Community Medicine,** Mumbai, v. 33, n.´, p. 15-18, 2008.

HARTUNG, D. M.; TOCHETTE, D. OverView of clinical research design. **American Journal of Health-System Pharmacy,** Bethesda, v. 66, n. 4, p. 398-408, 2009.
HECK, M. R.; KANTORSKI, L. P.; BORGES, A. M.; LOPES, C. V.; SANTOS, M. C.; PINHO, L. B. Actions taken by professionals at a psychosocial care centre when dealing with users who have attempted or are at risk of suicide. **Texto Contexto de Enfermagem,** Florianópolis, v. 21, n. 1, p. 26 - 33, 2012.

JOE, S.; DANIEL, D. R.; PATRICK, E. J. Suicide acceptability is related to suicide planning in U.S. adolescents and young adults. **Suicide and Life Threatening Behaviour,** New York, v. 37, n. 2, p. 165-178, 2007.

JUNG, J. H.; OLSON, D. V. A. Religion, stress, and suicide acceptability in south korea. Social forces, a scientific medium of social study and interpretation, **Chapei Hill,** Baltimore, v. 92, n. 3, p. 1039- 1059, 2014.

KANTORSKI, L. P.; CAVADA, C.; OLIVEIRA, C.; HAUFFEN, F. Serviço de atenção diária de saúde mental - um espaço de diálogo entre a universidade e os serviços. **Revista de Saúde URCAMP,** Bagé, v. 4, n. 1, p. 74 - 82, 2000.

KARMAN, P.; KOOL, N.; POSLAWSKY, I. E.; MEIJEL, B. V. Nurses' attitudes towards self-harm: a literature review. **Journal of Psychiatric and Mental Health Nursing,** Boston, v. 22, p. 65-75, 2015.

KELLY, M; MCCARTHY, S; SAHM, L. J. Krowledge, attitudes and beliefs of patients and carers regarding medication adherence: a review of qualitative literature. **European Journal of Clinical Pharmacology,** Berlin, v. 70, n. 12, p. 1423-31, 2014.

KAPLAN, H. L; SADOCK, B.; GREBB, J. **Compendium of psychiatry:** behavioural sciences and clinical psychiatry. 7 ed. Porto Alegre: Artes Médicas, 2002.

LARKIN, G. L.; SMITH, R. P.; BEAUTRAIS, A. L. Trends in US emergency department visits for suicide attempts, 1992 - 2001. **The Journal of Crisis Intervention and Suicide Prevention,** London, v. 92, n. 2, p. 73-80, 2008.

MCCARTHY, L.; GIJBELS, H. An examination of emergency department nurses' attitudes towards deliberate self-harm in an Irish teaching hospital. **International Emergency Nursing,** Oxford, v. 18, n. 1, p. 29-35, 2010.

MEADOWS, K. A. So you want to do research? 4: an introduction to quantitative methods. **British journal of community nursing,** England, v. 8, n. 11, p. 519- 526, 2003.
MENON, V. Suicide risk assessment and formulation: An update. **Asian Journal of Psychiatry,** Amsterdam, v. 6, n. 5, p. 430-435, 2013.

NANTON, E. The definition of assisted suicide. **Anglican Journal,** Toronto, v. 140, n. 1, p. 6, 2014. Available at : http://go.galegroup.com/ps/i.do?id=GALE%7CA355867615&v=2.1&u=capes&it=r&p= AONE&sw=w&asid=a2dc5c762004d2ccb4c297df42a3d19e Accessed: 11 May 2016.

NEBHINANI, M.; NEBHIMANI, N.; TAMPHASANA, L.; GAIKWAD A. D. Nursing students' attitude towards suicide attempters: A study from rural part of northern India. **Journal Neurosciences in Rural Practice,** Mumbai, v. 4, n. 4, p. 400-407, 2013.

NORHEIM, A. B.; GRIMHOLT, T. K.; LOSKUTOVA, E.; EKEBERG, O. Attitudes towards suicidal behaviour among professionals at mental health outpatient clinics in Stavropol, Russia and Oslo, Norway. **BioMed Central Psychiatric,** London, v. 16, n. 268, p. 2-12, 2016.

OESEBURG, B.; HILBERTS, R.; ROODBOL, P. P. Essential competencies for the education of nursing assistants and care helpers in elderly care, **Health Services Research,** Scotland, v. 35, n. 10, p. 32-35, 2015.

WORLD HEALTH ORGANISATION (OMS). **World report on violence and health.** Geneva: WHO; 2002.

WORLD HEALTH ORGANISATION (OMS). **Suicide prevention: a resource for counsellors a resource for counsellors.** World Health Organisation - WHO: Geneva, 2006.

OSAFO, J.; KNIZEK, B. L.; AKOTIA, C. S.; HJELMELAND, H. Attitudes of psychologists and nurses toward suicide and suicide prevention in Ghana: A qualitative study. **International Journal of Nursing Studies,** Dubai, v. 49, n. 6, p. 691-700, 2012.

OWENS, D.; HORROCKS, J.; HOUSE, A. Fatal and non-fatal repetition of self-harm. Systematic review. **British Journal of Psychiatry,** n. 181, p. 193-199, 2002.
PALLANT, J. **SPSS Survival Manual:** a step by step guide to data analysis using SPSS. 4th ed. Berkshire: McGraw-Hill, 2010.

PATTERSON, P.; WHITTINGTON, R.; BOGG, J. Measuring nurse attitudes towards deliberate self-harm: the self-harm antipathy scale (SHAS). **Journal of Psychiatric and Mental Health Nursing,** Oxford, v. 14, n. 5, p. 438-445, 2007.

PINTO-FOLTZ, M. D.; LOGSDON, M. C. Reducing stigma relating to mental disorders: initiatives, interventions and recommendations for nursing. **Archives of Psychiatric Nursing,** Orlando, v. 23, n.1, p. 32-40, 2009.

POLIT, D.; BECK, C. T.; HUNGLER, B. **Fundamentals of nursing research: methods, evaluation and utilisation. 6.** ed. Porto Alegre: Artmed, 2011.

POREDDI, V.; THIMMAIAH, R.; RAMU, R.; SELVI, S.; GANDHI, S.; MATH, S. B. Gender Differences Related to Attitudes Toward Suicide and Suicidal Behaviour. **Community Mental Health Journal,** Lexington, v. 52, n. 2, p. 228-232, 2016.

QUEVEDO, J.; SCHMITT, R.; KAPCZINSKI, F. **Emergências Psiquiátricas.** 2 ed. Porto Alegre: Artmed, 2008.440 p.

RAMBERG, I.; LUCCA, M. A. D.; HADLACZKY, G. the impact of knowledge of suicide prevention and work experience among clinicai staff cn attitudes towards working with suicidai patients and suicide prevention. **International Journal of Environmental Research and Public Health,** Basel, 2016, v. 13, n. 195, p. 1-12, 2016.

REGISTERED NURSES' ASSOCIATION OF ONTARIO (RNAO) **Nursing Best Practice Guideline:** Assessment and Care of Adults at Risk for Suicidal Ideation and Behaviour. RNAO: Ontario, 2009.

REUTER, E.; CAMBA, J. D. Understanding emergency workers' behaviour and perspectives on design and safety in the workplace. **Applied Ergonomics,** London, v. 59, p. 73-83, 2017.

ROTHES, I. A.; HENRIQUES, M. R.; LEAL, J. B.; LEMOS, M. S. facing a patient who seeks help after a suicide attempt: the difficulties of health professionals. **Crisis,** Porto, v. 35, n. 2, p. 110-122, 2014.
SAUNDERS, K. E. A.; HAWNTON, K. FORTUNE, S.; FARRELL, S. Attitudes and knowledge of clinicai staff regarding people who self-harm: a systematic review. **Journal of Affective Disorders,** Amsterdam, v. 139, n. 3, p. 205-216, 2012.

SPINO, E.; KAMEG, K. M.; CLINE, T. W.; TERHORST, L.; MITCHELL, A. M. Impact of social support on symptoms of depression and loneliness in survivors bereaved by suicide. **Archives of Psychiatric Nursing,** Orlando, v. 30, n. 5, p. 602-606, 2016.

SANTOS, M. S.; COIMBRA, V. C. C.; RIBEIRO, J. P. Attending emergency psychiatric held by the nurse of the Service mobile emergency. **Revista de Enfermagem UFPE Online,** Pelotas, v. 5, n. 9, p. 2197- 2205, 2011.

SIMON, A. E.; SCHOENDORF, K. C. Emergency department visits for mental health conditions among us children, 2001-2011. **Clinical Paediatrics,** Philadelphia, v. 53, n.14, p. 1359-1366, 2014.

SCOCCO, P.; TOFFORL, E.; PILOTTO, E.; PERTILE, R. Psychiatrists' emotional reactions to patient suicide behaviour. **Journal of Psychiatric Practice,** Philadelphia, v. 18, n. 2, p. 94-108,2012.

SILVERMAN, M. M.; BERMAN, A. L.; SANDDAL, N. D.; O'CARROL, P. W.; JOINER, T. E. rebuilding the tower of babel: a revised nomenclature for the study of suicide and suicidal behaviours. Part 2: suiciderelated ideations, communications, and behaviours. **Suicide Life Threat Behavior,** New York, v. 37, n. 3, p. 264-277, 2007.

SOUSA, V.; DRIESSNACK, M.; MENDES, I. A. C. Review of research designs relevant to nursing. Part 1: Quantitative Research Designs. **Revista Latino-Americana de Enfermagem,** São Paulo, v. 15, n. 3, p. 1- 6, 2007.

SRIVASTAVA, M.; TIWARI, R. A comparative study of attitude of mental health versus non-mental professionals towards suicide indian. **Indian Journal of Psychological Medicine,** Mumbai, v. 34, n. 1, p. 66-69, 2012.

SUN, M. K.; BAEK, J. H.; HAN, D. H.; LEE, Y. S.; YURGELUN-TODD, D. A. Psychosocial - Environmental risk factors for suicide attempts in adolescents with suicidal ideation: findings from a sample of 73,238 adolescents. **Suicide and Life-Threatening Behaviour,** Korea, v. 45, n. 4, p. 477-487, 2015.

SUOMINEN, K.; SUOKAS, J.; LÕNNQVIST, J. Attitudes of general hospital emergency room personnel towards attempted suicide patients. **Nordic Journal of Psychiatry,** Oslo, v. 61, n. 5, p. 387-392, 2007.

TALSETH, A. G.; GILJE, F. Unburdening suffering: responses of psychiatrists to patients' suicide deaths. **Nursing Ethics,** London, v. 14, n. 5, p. 620-636, 2007. Available at: <http://www.ncbi.nlm.nih.gov/pubmed/17901173>. Accessed on: 15 June 2016.

VANNOY, S. D.; TAI-SEALE, M.; DUBERSTEIN, P.; EATON, L. J.; COOK, M. A. Suicide ideation responses in late-life primary care. **Journal of General Internal Medicine,** v. 26, n. 9, p. 1005-11, 2011.

VIEIRA, S. **Introduction to biostatistics.** Rio de Janeiro: Elsevier, 2008.

VIDAL, C. E. L.; GONTIJO, E. D. Suicide attempts and reception in emergency services: the perception of those who attempt it. **Cadernos de Saúde Coletiva,** Rio de Janeiro, v. 21, n. 2, p. 108-14, 2013.

VOLPE, F. M.; CORRÊA, H.; BARRERO, S. P. **Epidemiology of suicide.** In: CORRÊA, H.; PEREZ, S. (Orgs.). Suicide, a preventable death. São Paulo: Atheneu, 2006. p. 11-27.

WERLANG, B. G.; BOTEGA, N. J. **Comportamento suicida.** Porto Alegre: Artmed, 2004.

WHEATLEY, M.; AUSTIN-PAYNE, H. Nursing staff knowledge and attitudes towards deliberate self-harm in adults and adolescents in an inpatien: setting. **Behavioural and Cognitive Psychotherapy,** New York, v. 37, p. 293-309, 2009.

WORLD HEALTH ORGANISATION (WHO). The World Health Report 2001. **Mental Health:** new understanding, newhope. Geneva, 2001.

WORLD HEALTH ORGANISATION (WHO). **Prevention of mental disorders:** effective interventions and policy options. Geneva, 2004.

WORLD HEALTH ORGANISATION (WHO). **Suicide prevention:** facing the challenges, building Solutions. European Ministerial Conference on Mental Heath 2005 (January): 1- 6.

WORLD HEALTH ORGANISATION (WHO). WHO/HEN Multicentre Study. **Crisis,** Porto, v. 27, n.1, p. 4- 15, 2006.
WORLD HEALTH ORGANISATION (WHO). **Preventing suicide.** A resource for media professionals. Geneva: World Health Organisation, 2008.

WORLD HEALTH ORGANISATION (WHO). Preventing suicide - A global imperative. 2014.
Available at   :
<http://apps.who. i nt/i ris/bitstream/10665/131056/1 /9789241564779_eng.pdf?ua=1 &u a=1>.
Accessed on: 11 September 2015.

YIP, P. S. F.; CAINE, E.; YOUSUF, S.; CHANG, S. S.; WU, K. C. C; CHEN, Y. Y. Means restriction for suicide prevention. **Lancet,** New York, v.379, n. 9834, p. 2393- 2399, 2012.

XIAOHIU, Z.; TAO, L.; XIA, H.; YINAN, J.; CAO, N. Barrier of emergency departments in providing mental health services for patients with suicide attempts. **Journal of Chinese Medicine,** Hong Kong, v. 95, n. 23, p. 1833-1836, 2015.

ZADRAVEC, T.; GRAD, O. Origins of suicidality: compatibility of layand expert belirfs - Qualitative study. **Pshychiatria Danubina,** Croatia, v. 25, n. 2, p.152-155, 2013.

ZANI, A.V.; NOGUEIRA, M. S. Incidentes críticos do processo ensino-aprendizagem do curso de graduação em enfermagem, segundo a percepção de alunos e docentes. **Revista Latinoamericana de Enfermagem,** São Paulo, v. 14, n. 5, p. 742-748, 2006.

Appendices
Appendix A: Informed consent form for research participants

Dear Nursing Professional,

We hereby invite you to take part in the project entitled ***"Meaning of suicide, attitudes and impacts experienced by nursing professionals working in emergencies", the*** general aim of which is to understand the meanings of suicide for nursing professionals working in emergencies.

Your participation may involve two stages. In the first stage we will ask you to help us answer the self-administered questionnaire on attitudes towards suicidal behaviour, which takes approximately 10 minutes to complete. You may also be invited to take part in the second stage, which will be an audio-recorded interview with open questions about your professional experiences related to suicide and what you think about this subject. The interview will take between 30 and 40 minutes. The interview will take place in a private location and will be scheduled so as not to jeopardise your work. We therefore ask for your cooperation and authorisation to answer the questionnaire and, if necessary, take part in the interview. Your identity will be kept confidential and, at the end of the study, only the results will be published in the various media (such as scientific journals). Your participation in this research will not be paid for and will not cost you any money.

If you need to, you can contact us for any reason, including to stop taking part in the research at any time, without any harm being caused to you by the researchers. We undertake to provide any additional information and clarification if you have any questions about the research. In this case, you can contact the researchers by telephone on (16) 33153439 or by e-mail: kellygiacchero@eerp.usp.br and dfmagrini@yahoo.com.br and the EERP Research Ethics Committee by telephone on (16) 3315 3386 or at Av. Bandeirantes 3900 from Monday to Friday from 8am to 5pm. The purpose of the Ethics Committee is to guarantee that human rights are upheld and that research participants are ethically protected. It evaluates research at all stages of studies involving human beings, from the preparation of the project to the final report. We would like to emphasise that this research was approved by the CEP-EERP.

You have the right to compensation should any damage occur as a result of your participation in the research, on the part of the researcher and the institutions involved in the different phases of the research. The risks and/or discomfort of participating in the study are minimal and are related to the time taken for the interview and the discomfort of answering some questions. To minimise these issues, we may listen to you, talk about something else or interrupt the interview, according to your needs. Your participation could bring benefits in terms of improving care for clients with suicidal behaviour.

If you agree to take part in this research, you will do so voluntarily and you must sign this consent form in two copies, one of which will remain with you. Thank you in advance and we are at your disposal for any questions.

Kelly Graziani Giacchero Vedana	Daniel Fernando Magrini
Researcher responsible	Guiding student

I declare that I have been duly informed about the research and the procedures involved and I agree to take part in this study. I have received a copy of this informed consent form and have been given the opportunity to read it and clarify my doubts.

Location:_______________//. _________________________________
Participant's signature

Appendix B: Script for collecting sociodemographic data

1. Gender: ( ) 1. Female ( ) 2. Male
Service: ( ) I.UEfTrauma ( ) 2.UE/SEC ( ) 3.HC/BOX ( ) 4.EU/Psychiatry ( )5.SAMU
2. Position: ( ) 1. Nurse ( ) 2.Nursing Technician ( ) 3. Nursing assistant.
3. Date of birth: / / Date of interview: / /
4. Education: ( ) I.Technical/Vocational ( ) 2.Higher education incomplete ( ) 3.Complete university degree ( ) 4.Specialisation/Residency ( )5.Master's degree ( ) 6. Doctorate
5.Do you have specific training in Mental Health? ( ) 1. Yes ( ) 2. No
6. Length of time in nursing (complete years):
7. Length of time working in the ward (complete years):
8. Have you ever worked in a psychiatric or mental health service? ( ) 1. yes ( )

2. No

If yes, for how long (approximately)? _________________ years or ______ months

9. Have you ever received specific training on suicide? ( ) 1. Yes ( ) 2. No

If yes, for how long (approximately)?   _______ years or
_____ months

Annexes

ANNEX A - Authorisation from the Research Ethics Committee of the Ribeirão Preto School of Nursing of the University of São Paulo

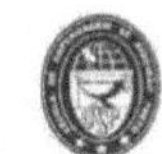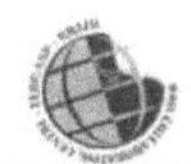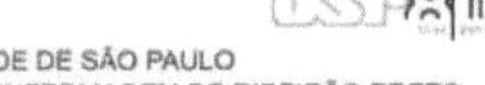

UNIVERSIDADE DE SÃO PAULO
ESCOLA DE ENFERMAGEM DE RIBEIRÃO PRETO

Centro Colaborador da Organização Mundial de Saúde
para o Desenvolvimento da Pesquisa em Enfermagem

Avenida Bandeirantes, 3900 - Ribeirão Preto - São Paulo - Brasil - CEP 14040-902
Fone: 55 16 3315-3392 - 55 16 3315-3391 - Fax 55 16 3315-0518
www.eerp.usp.br - eerp@eerp.usp.br

COMITÊ DE ÉTICA EM PESQUISA DA EERP/USP

Of.CEP-EERP/USP – 028/2015

Ribeirão Preto, 4 de março de 2015.

Prezada Senhora,

Comunicamos que o projeto de pesquisa, abaixo especificado, foi analisado e considerado **APROVADO AD REFERENDUM** pelo Comitê de Ética em Pesquisa da Escola de Enfermagem de Ribeirão Preto da Universidade de São Paulo, em 4 de março de 2015.

Protocolo CAAE: 40072214.0.0000.5393

Projeto: Significados do suicídio, atitudes e impactos experimentados por profissionais de enfermagem que atuam em emergências.

Pesquisadores: Kelly Graziani Giacchero Vedana

Em atendimento à Resolução 466/12, deverá ser encaminhado ao CEP o relatório final da pesquisa e a publicação de seus resultados, para acompanhamento, bem como comunicada qualquer intercorrência ou a sua interrupção.

Atenciosamente,

Profa. Dra. Claudia Benedita dos Santos
Coordenadora do CEP-EERP/USP

Ilma. Sra.
Profa. Dra. Kelly Graziani Giacchero Vedana
Departamento de Enfermagem Psiquiátrica e Ciências Humanas
Escola de Enfermagem de Ribeirão Preto - USP

ANNEX B - Questionnaire on Attitudes towards Suicidal Behaviour

QUESTIONÁRIO DE ATITUDES EM RELAÇÃO AO COMPORTAMENTO SUICIDA

Este questionário pesquisa atitudes em relação ao **comportamento suicida**.

Evite pensar demais para responder. Estamos interessados em sua resposta espontânea, a primeira idéia que lhe ocorrer, sem se preocupar se é "certo" ou "errado".

Algumas informações solicitadas logo abaixo permitirão criar um código. Desse modo, você não será identificado quando analisarmos os dados. Por favor, use LETRA DE FORMA.

Agradecemos sua participação.

Ao responder as questões, **assinale com um traço** a posição que mais se aproximar de sua opinião. Veja nos exemplos abaixo:

EXEMPLOS

"EU GOSTO DE OUVIR MÚSICA SERTANEJA"

| Discordo totalmente | | Concordo plenamente |

A resposta acima indica concordância com a proposição, mas não uma concordância total. A concordância total seria indicada por um traço ao final da linha, como abaixo:

| Discordo totalmente | | Concordo plenamente |

Se, em relação à afirmativa, você não tiver opinião formada ou for indiferente, assinale no centro da linha, como indicado:

| Discordo totalmente | | Concordo plenamente |

1. Sinto-me capaz de ajudar uma pessoa que tentou se matar

| Discordo totalmente | | Concordo plenamente |

2. Quem fica a ameaçar, geralmente não se mata

| Discordo totalmente | | Concordo plenamente |

3. Apesar de tudo, penso que, se uma pessoa deseja se matar, ela tem esse direito

Discordo   ____   Concordo
totalmente   plenamente

4. Diante de um suicídio penso: se alguém tivesse conversado, a pessoa teria encontrado outro caminho

Discordo   ____   Concordo
totalmente   plenamente

5. No fundo, prefiro não me envolver muito com pacientes que tentaram o suicídio

Discordo   ____   Concordo
totalmente   plenamente

6. A vida é um dom de Deus, e só Ele pode tirar

Discordo   ____   Concordo
totalmente   plenamente

7. Sinto-me capaz de perceber quando um paciente tem risco de se matar

Discordo   ____   Concordo
totalmente   plenamente

8. Geralmente, quem se mata tem alguma doença mental

Discordo   ____   Concordo
totalmente   plenamente

9. Tenho receio de perguntar sobre idéias de suicídio, e acabar induzindo o paciente a isso

Discordo   ____   Concordo
totalmente   plenamente

10. Tenho preparo profissional para lidar com pacientes com risco de suicídio

Discordo   ____   Concordo
totalmente   plenamente

11. É preciso ter certa dose de coragem para se matar

Discordo   ____   Concordo
totalmente   plenamente

12. Sinto-me inseguro(a) para cuidar de pacientes com risco de suicídio

Discordo   ____   Concordo
totalmente   plenamente

13. No fundo, às vezes dá até raiva, porque tanta gente querendo viver... e aquele paciente querendo morrer

14. Se eu sugerir uma interconsulta psiquiátrica para um paciente que falou em se matar, penso que isso será bem aceito pelo seu médico assistente

Discordo ____ Concordo
totalmente plenamente

15. A gente se sente impotente diante de uma pessoa que quer se matar

Discordo ____ Concordo
totalmente plenamente

16. Quem tem Deus no coração, não vai tentar se matar

Discordo ____ Concordo
totalmente plenamente

17. No caso de pacientes que estejam sofrendo muito devido a uma doença física, acho mais aceitável a idéia de suicídio

Discordo ____ Concordo
totalmente plenamente

18. Quando uma pessoa fala de por fim à vida, tento tirar aquilo da cabeça dela

Discordo ____ Concordo
totalmente plenamente

19. Quem quer se matar mesmo, não fica "tentando" se matar

Discordo ____ Concordo
totalmente plenamente

20. Um paciente internado dificilmente se mata sem que tenha um forte motivo pra isso

Discordo ____ Concordo
totalmente plenamente

21. Eu já passei por situações que me fizeram pensar em cometer suicídio

Discordo ____ Concordo
totalmente plenamente

Obrigado por sua colaboração!

ANNEX C - Authorisation to use the "Questionnaire on Attitudes towards Suicidal Behaviour"

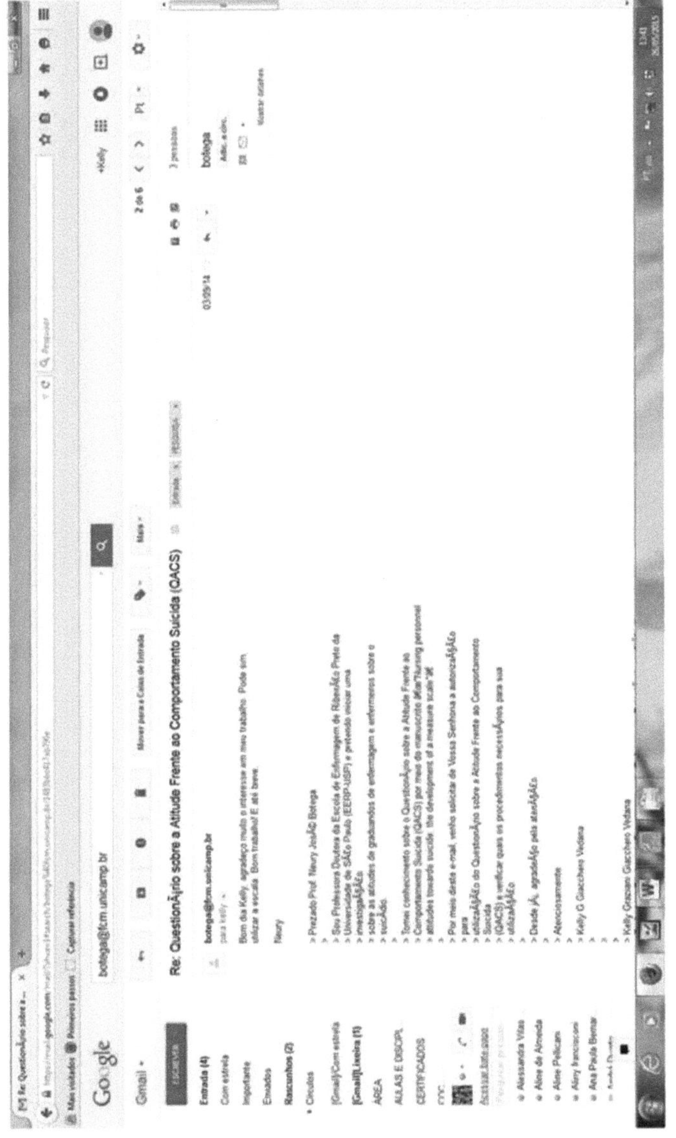

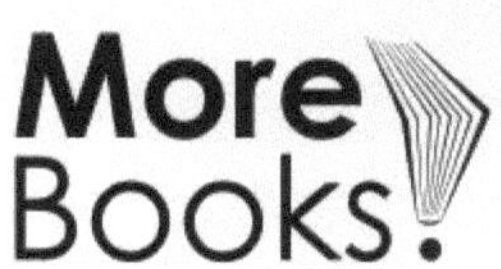

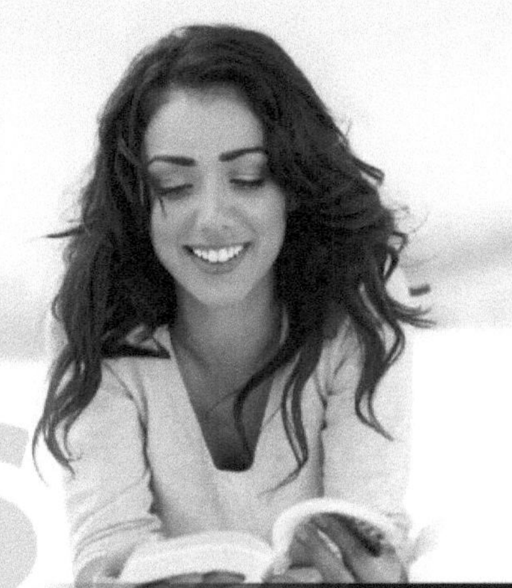

I want morebooks!

Buy your books fast and straightforward online - at one of world's fastest growing online book stores! Environmentally sound due to Print-on-Demand technologies.

Buy your books online at
www.morebooks.shop

Kaufen Sie Ihre Bücher schnell und unkompliziert online – auf einer der am schnellsten wachsenden Buchhandelsplattformen weltweit! Dank Print-On-Demand umwelt- und ressourcenschonend produziert.

Bücher schneller online kaufen
www.morebooks.shop

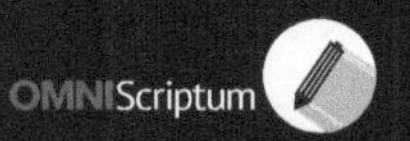

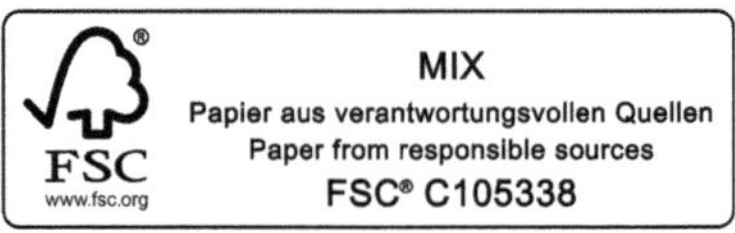

Printed by Books on Demand GmbH, Norderstedt / Germany